D1728161

The Witch as Psychopomp

Text © Sharon Day, 2022

Cover Design and interior typesetting © Nuno Moreira, 2022

Images © Nuno Moreira, and Public Domain

Library of Congress Cataloguing-in-Publication Data ISBN 978-1-913023-09-6

www.roseankhpublishing.com
www.instagram.com/roseankhpublishing
www.facebook.com/roseankhpublishing
www.twitter.com/RA_Publishing

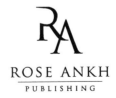

ROSE ANKH
PUBLISHING

Dr Elisabeth Kübler-Ross meets Dion Fortune
at Maxine Sanders' Temple of the Mother

The Witch as Psychopomp

Sharon Day

Also by Sharon Day

'Through the Veil of the Digital Revolution and into the Abyss of Artificial Intelligence: The Insidious Desensitisation of Humanity' in *A Shadow Within: Evil in Fantasy and Science Fiction*, Edited by Francesca Barbini, Luna Press Publishing, Edinburgh, 2019

Author's Note

"What shall we put as your occupation?" I asked the iconic Maxine Sanders, popularly known as the Witch Queen of the late '60s and 70s.

The year was 2017 and we were completing the routine business of setting up *alexandrianwitchcraft.org*, the online archive of what today is known as the Alexandrian tradition of Witchcraft, one founded by her and her late husband Alex, popularly dubbed 'King of the Witches.'

"Bereavement Counsellor", she replied without any hesitation...

Of all the answers she might have given, this one was unexpected and yet came as no surprise, for it coincided neatly with a talk I was due to give several months later at an academic conference - 'Death, Dying and Disposal 13' in 2017 - at the University of Central Lancashire. That talk forms the substance of the present booklet. It provoked many questions and comments from members of the audience at the time, among them a funeral undertaker who kindly remarked that the notions advanced were 'a breath of fresh air'. My hope is that readers may find them equally bracing.

The Coven of the Stag King came into being at the Summer Solstice of 2015 with Maxine Sanders consenting to serve it as guide and mentor. From the start, one of the questions we have asked candidates for initiation at the end of their instruction concerns their attitude to working with those close to death. This is because part of our work includes easing the process of transition - and by that I don't mean what's nowadays called "assisted dying" - from this life to the one that we believe comes after it.

The Witch as Psychopomp*

Dr Elisabeth Kübler-Ross

meets Dion Fortune

at Maxine Sanders'

Temple of the Mother

Sharon Day

* from the Greek term "Guider of Souls", a reference to those,
usually benevolent spirits or angels, committed to guiding the dead
from this world into the next.

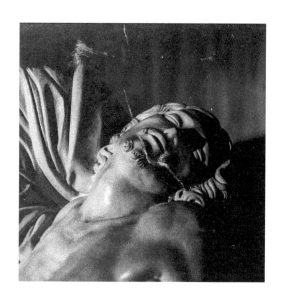

The Nexus

The year 1969 was a significant one for two remarkable women, one a Swiss-American doctor, the other an English witch. In that year Dr Elisabeth Kübler-Ross, the Swiss-American psychiatrist summarised the dying process in the 'Five Stages of Grief' model set out in her seminal work *On Death and Dying*. The challenges she encountered prior to its release and even more so in the wake of it, came mainly from doctors and academics, sceptical, even distrustful, of her pioneering work with the dying. It would be a running theme throughout her subsequent career. Today, thanks to her resilience and impassioned commitment, Dr Kübler-Ross is acknowledged as the forerunner of the worldwide hospice movement.

In the year of the book's publication and on the other side of the Atlantic, Maxine Sanders, too, found herself in the public eye. Thrust to the forefront of the nascent revival of witchcraft, she was on that account ridiculed, derided, and, on one occasion, stoned on the streets of Manchester, her home in the north of England. And all because, the popular press had exposed her as a practising witch. Missing from view, then and subsequently, were the depth and commitment of the work being undertaken by the healing coven she went on to establish in the mid-70s, dubbed The Temple of the Mother. And that work included a service to the dying that was, in purpose if not in expression, no different from that of Dr. Kubler-Ross.

Both women had identified a glaring failure in our duty of care to the dying, at the time a taboo subject. In her own work with the dying, Maxine Sanders parallelled that of Kübler-Ross, even if its forms of expression were different. These were incorporated in the rites and practice of her Temple of the Mother. They include a Sending Forth Rite, which I shall return to later, and

were grounded in the teachings
of the influential occultist, Dion
Fortune, who died in 1946.

In its approach, what has since
become known as the Craft of the
Wise takes into sympathetic account
the preferences, religious, cultural
and social, of the dying person. The
aim is a collaborative undertaking
in which he or she can accept, even
embrace, the transition towards what,
we believe, is the final Mystery of life,
a portal to the next phase of our human
experience. Needless to say, the
preferences, religious or practical, of
the dying person are fully respected
throughout the procedure, while
the participation of his or her loved
ones is welcomed.

The aims of Dr Kübler-Ross and her promotion of the hospice movement are by now realised in countless death doula and hospice training courses. In substance they differ little from what happens in their magical equivalent, the latter involving visualisation and meditation and what is known as pathworking. The language may differ but the meaning and purpose do not. In witchcraft they begin with the contemplation of one's own mortality, the first question asked of everyone is, what it is we fear about dying?

According to Dion Fortune there are two answers: the unknown and separation from our loved ones. A third suggestion by Caitlin Doughty, an American mortician, author of the book *Smoke Gets in Your Eyes* and founder of the Order of the Good Death, is dread of the dissolution of the body.

Securing an understanding of what, in our view as occultists, happens to the immortal part of us - soul, spirit or whatever - during and after the dying process is held to facilitate a fruitful collaboration with the dying and their loved ones, offering both reassurance, comfort, and peace of mind. In going about it, however, we take scrupulous care not to impose our own views on the dying or their family about the precise nature of the afterlife. We are adamant that our work is not about securing a deathbed conversion!

On the contrary, a member of the Temple of the Mother recently wrote to me of her many years working in a children's hospice in Wales:

Individual cultures and wishes have to be first and foremost. However, one can set the right conditions and environment to allow the passing to be fulfilling and complete. Creating a safe, secure, warm, informed environment, providing support, allows them to feel in control of the death, which can make a big difference to the person experiencing the death and the family in their bereavement. Any inner work should be done with this in mind with full respect and care.

Dion Fortune reduces death, or as she terms it 'the Great Anaesthetist', to its fundamental components: natural and violent. The difference is that natural death takes place gradually, with the soul easing itself from the body like a child's milk tooth rather being yanked out by the dentist. In short, death is either peaceful or not.

The person who sees death coming has the opportunity to consider what, if anything, to expect, should he survive the event. However pessimistic about post-mortem survival, he will at least be prepared for that possibility and, as a result, accept it when it happens. The same is true of someone confident of survival who meets a sudden or accidental death. Both will be ready to submit to what Tibetan Buddhism calls the 'Surrender of Consciousness'.

By contrast a death that is sudden or unpeaceful, the latter involving a sustained conflict with the Great Anaesthetist, may involve a less peaceful or less confident transition. And here, witches believe, we may be privileged to offer help and guidance, specifically by recruiting entities known as the Beings of Light. I shall have more to say about these later.

Just as the newborn child may arrive at the Gates of Life "normally", by which I mean head-first, or "abnormally", that is, feet first, so in our belief should a dying person ideally quit this mortal life, head - by which I mean his higher levels of consciousness - first, leaving the rest of him to follow. On this I shall have more to say later.

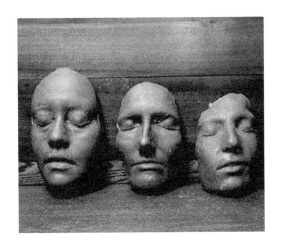

Setting the Right Conditions

In order to provide maximum
assistance to the dying, the witch-
as-psychopomp develops an
individual technique for 'parking'
- that is temporarily suspending
- his or her "ego" or, if you prefer,
self-centred consciousness. This can
best be described in terms of either
empathy or telepathy, the difference
being that the empath is sensitive
to - even shares - the emotions of
others, while the telepath perceives
those emotions dispassionately and
bereft of any emotional attachment.

Not that the second of these necessarily precludes compassion. Either approach can be fruitful.

The first step is to rid oneself of one's 'I', counterintuitive though that is to our natural disposition. In part this is because it would otherwise frustrate our wish to say or do something specifically meaningful for the dying or their family, but above all because its removal in turn removes our own instinctive fear of dying. After all, when we contemplate someone on their deathbed, it is a stark reminder of what's also in store for us, the only uncertainty being the how and the when.

Temporarily detaching - or, if you like, "parking" - our self-consciousness or, perhaps more correctly, our *self-centeredness* is a matter of technique. A medium of my acquaintance remembers nothing at all of what she says while entranced so takes care to record her sessions for her client's benefit as much as her own. Once, she was asked what she does with her consciousness when a session with a client is in progress. *'Oh, we go for a cup of tea,'* was her reply. Funnily enough, I've noticed that her newsfeed frequently contains images of cups of coffee or tea at whatever quirky cafe she happens to have visited. A living metaphor.

Both Dr Kübler-Ross and Maxine Sanders maintain that the dying

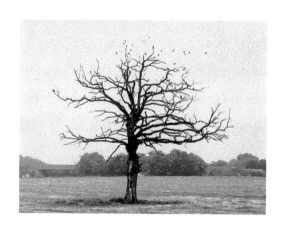

frequently express a wish to clear up 'unfinished business'. This may mean nothing more than the desire to have with them a listener by way of sounding board, not unlike the final confession our Catholic friends hope to make before dying. Personally, I liken my job to that of an airport check-in agent, the dying person being the traveller with too much baggage on the scale. Unwilling to pay the excess, he discards a couple of bags or a suitcase and immediately lightens the load. At times the sympathetic presence of another human may be all that's needed to lighten the load we all bear at the end of our lives. Often, too, the gentle touch of another's hand is reassurance enough.

Slipping the Moorings

The witch-as-psychopomp is equipped also to recognise the impediments or ties that can hold the soul back from advancing on its journey, not only during the process of dying but shortly after the event as well.

As a rule, children are better able to accept death than adults. Hospital wards and the prevailing camaraderie, even a touch of dark humour on occasion, seem to reconcile them to the inevitable, often in contrast to their parents whose desperate, if understandable, pleas that a mortally sick infant 'hang on' or 'keep fighting' risks tying them to a life they are ready to leave. Not infrequently an infant will take leave of life when his or her parent has briefly quit the bedside.

The dying adult, too, may be held back by ties or unfinished business, whether family disputes, inheritance issues, concerns about the welfare of loved ones in their absence - all of this goes back to the fear of separation from loved ones that Dion Fortune made much of in her work.

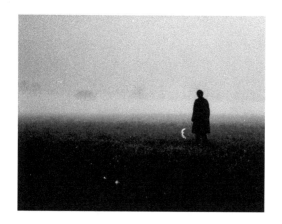

Ensuring a Point of No Return - Sealing the Body

No matter how much preparation is made for one's own death, anyone, even the most accomplished adept, can find living on the physical plane addictive and thus opt even after death to loiter in what had been familiar territory. This carries the risk of their being permanently earthbound. To prevent this, the body is ritually "sealed" through a series of banishings and invocations prior to committal. These encourage the soul to proceed on its way forwards.

Funeral

A funeral is for the living but
not unnoticed by the dead. We
have many accounts in which
the deceased, communicating
through mediums or psychics,
have described their funeral in
considerable detail. This accords
with a belief that the newly dead
enter a phase when, as if waking
from a deep sleep of death, they are
alert to what's happening here and
now before embarking on the next
stage of their journey.

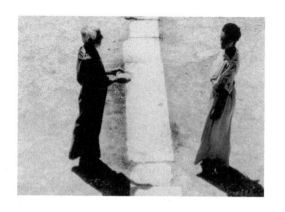

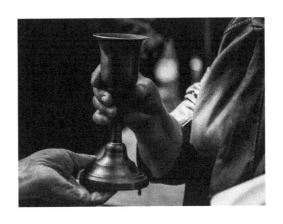

On the assumption that the 'Great Anaesthetist' has been left to do its work, the newly deceased wake up gently from their initial slumber, as if emerging from an induced sleep. Within our time frame this usually takes two weeks to happen, although it may vary from case to case. The time frame after a violent death is especially unpredictable, whereas in the wake of natural or what might be called "good" deaths, it happens sooner rather than later.

The role of the witch-as-psychopomp towards the living is to provide solace to those left behind to mourn, prompting, if appropriate, the release of any pent-up emotions and the tears that accompany them. Societal or cultural norms that inhibit the all-too human expression of grief, typified by the British 'stiff upper lip' or the myth that 'men don't cry' need to be sent packing, with mourners encouraged to acknowledge their loss and by so doing be reconciled to it. One must always welcome the first faint flutters of that phoenix which marks a new beginning, just as a barely perceptible quiver at one corner of someone's mouth augurs a smile soon to be reborn. That same smile signals the beginning of a healing process that will lead one day to renewed laughter and a reminder to the living that life is here to be lived. Lived for oneself and for others, indeed for Life itself.

Sending Forth Rite

The Sending Forth Rite was created by Maxine Sanders and the Temple of the Mother for deceased initiates. It is the means by which those deemed members of the Priesthood are safely and tenderly restored to the Womb of the Great Mother. One of its intentions is to forestall the possibility of a soul being bound to Earth, achieved by dissolving the 'etheric body' and allowing its physical counterpart to revert to its constituent elements.

On rare occasions, the same rite is used to send forth the troubled soul of non-initiates who might otherwise risk becoming earth-bound, causing distress not only to themselves but their surviving family as well.

One example might be that of a deceased mother overly concerned about the welfare of young children she has left behind, either alone or in the care of someone she fears may be unsuitable. Many such mothers cling to the earth plane until assured, if they ever can be, that all is indeed well.

Such in brief is the aim of the Sending Forth Rite - to provide reassurance and encouragement to those reluctant to embark on the posthumous voyage that awaits them.

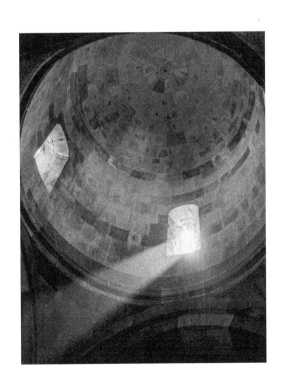

Violent, Sudden and Suicide Deaths - Bringing Forth the Non-denominational Beings of Light

Humanity is blessed by the companionship of Beings or, as they're sometimes called, "Angels" of Light, keen to assist and guide the newly deceased. They may, however, be thwarted in their efforts when a death was sudden, violent, or self-inflicted. Such a "tragic-death" soul risks becoming trapped within the moment of death, even unaware they have died or else forced to repeatedly relive the final moment of terror.

Our purpose is to break that cycle
and call upon the Beings of Light -
entities often present in hospitals,
war zones, and disaster sites -
to release these souls from their
torment and encourage them to
proceed on their posthumous way.

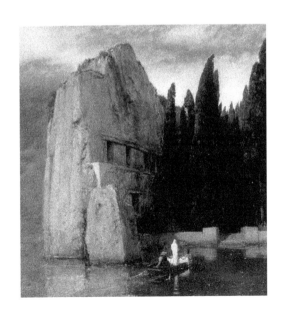

Suicide Rescue Circles

The primary ambition of a Suicide
Rescue Circle is to release an
unhappy soul from the shock of
their death, a failure to see beyond
the traumatic event they have
brought about. This work aims to
coax them into acknowledging their
new condition, putting behind them
the anger, sadness, sense of loss
or unfathomable distress that led
them to take their own life. To that
end, the Beings of Light mentioned
earlier are entreated to lend support
and take them forward.

Involved in this specific task are emotionally well-balanced witches with a long-term commitment to helping souls that are distressed or traumatised. It can be an extended process, not unlike most forms of therapy, with many meetings over a lengthy period, if appropriate. Commitment to it is akin to a formal contract: meeting times are fixed, each lasts for a prescribed length of time, and a scrupulous record of the proceedings is maintained. Questions addressed to the deceased entity will often provide information that can subsequently be verified, bringing added focus to the proceedings.

The group strives to entrap the negative energy still present, be it the product of fear, guilt, downright terror or, in some cases, a dark emptiness, and render it harmless. It can be a long and distressing process: one learns of the terrible ways people choose to end their life, while the emotional state leading to it is sometimes contagious, causing, unless due care is taken, physical or mental harm to one or more of the participants. Great effort is made, therefore, to take suitable precautions beforehand. Christians, both clergy and lay folk, sometimes undertake similar work and will, for example, recite the Lord's Prayer before and after it. We use what's called a banishing ritual to achieve the same result.

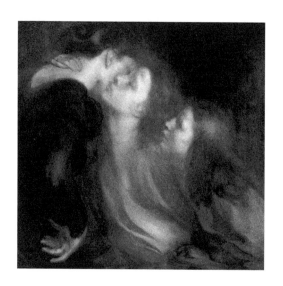

The reward for all this effort is less a sense of achievement than the perceptible joy of a deceased entity that has finally moved forwards into the Light.

Conclusion

If I had to sum up in one sentence why
those of us involved in Alexandrian
Witchcraft work with the dying and,
on occasion, the dead, it would be to
quote Patrick Swayze playing Sam
Wheat in the 1990 movie *Ghost*:
"It's amazing, Molly. The love
inside, you take it with you."

Afterword

A question put to me after delivering this talk was what might be the connection between Dr Kübler-Ross's investigation, towards the latter part of her life, of near- and after-death experiences, mediumship, and spiritualism on the one hand and Alexandrian Witchcraft on the other. This was something I'd not previously thought about but the answer came to me quite suddenly.

The emergence of the Kübler-Ross 'Five Stages of Grief' model coincided with the pioneering work undertaken by Maxine Sanders, who at that time was following an approach to Witchcraft incorporating the teachings of the renowned occultist, Dion Fortune, herself, a qualified psychotherapist. It may be no coincidence therefore that the Kübler-Ross approach to dying similarly accords with what Dion Fortune described in her book, *Through the Gates of Death*. In it the author, who died in 1946 describes the stages through which a soul passes on its final journey from this world to the next. In addition, she too, suggests how others might assist it in the process.

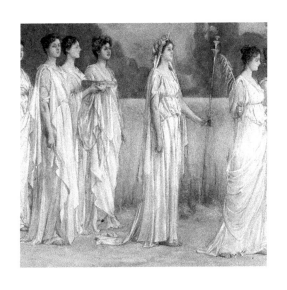

Notes on Sources

Anfara Jr, Vincent A. and Mertz,
Norma T, editors. *Theoretical
Frameworks in Qualitative Research*,
Thousand Oaks: Sage Publications,
Inc., 2006.

Doughty, Caitlin. *Smoke Gets In
Your Eyes*, Edinburgh: Canongate
Books, 2016.

Doughty, Caitlin. Founder of *The
Order of the Good Death*,

Los Angeles, California:
www.orderofthegooddeath.com.

Kübler-Ross, Elisabeth M.D. *On Death
& Dying*, New York: Scribner, 2014.

Kübler-Ross, Elisabeth M.D. *Is
there Life after Death?*, available at
www.audible.co.uk (Release Date:
23 Nov 2015).

Rinpoche, Sogyal. *Living Well, Dying
Well*, available at www.audible.co.uk
(Release Date: 3 Nov 2015).

Sanders, Maxine. *Fire Child*, Oxford: Mandrake of Oxford, 2008.

Society of the Inner Light. *Dion Fortune's Through the Gates of Death and Spiritualism in the Light of Occult Science*, Wellingborough: The Aquarian Press, 1987.

Weaver, Matt. "Patrick Swayze's last TV interview: 'Love- it's the one thing you can take with you when you die.'" *The Guardian*, Tuesday 15 September, 2009.

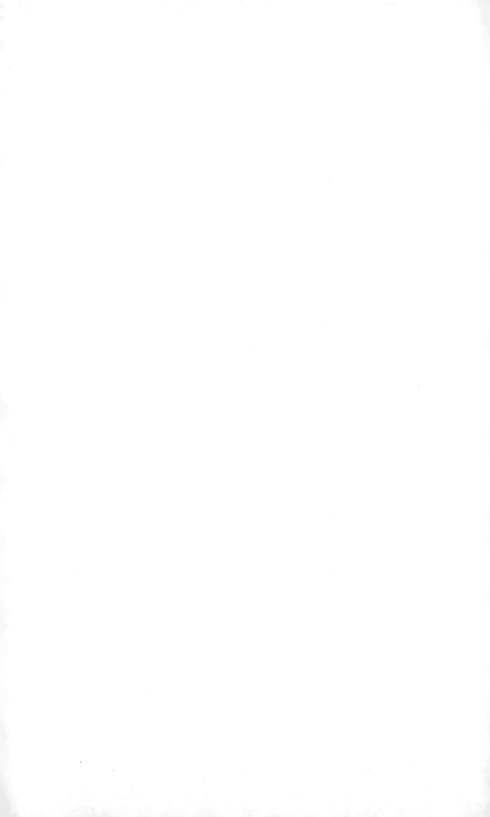

About the Author

American by birth and British by marriage, Sharon's academic career began with one year in Japan as an exchange student in 1980. She would return there for college and after having graduated from law school in New York City in 1992, with her husband, also a lawyer, when he took up a post in Tokyo years later.

After repatriating to London in 1997, Sharon felt drawn to esotericism and the occult, subsequently discovering what she felt was a vocation within Alexandrian witchcraft. Her search for suitable training and practical experience took her from London to Australia, the United States, and finally back to London, where she became the personal student of Maxine Sanders, co-founder of the Alexandrian Tradition.

Today, she leads the Coven of the Stag King in London under the eldership - and discreet guidance of Maxine.

Sharon is also the founder of Rose Ankh Publishing Ltd, a book publisher of unique occult, historical, philosophical, and biographical works, including volumes which are considered 'lost' due to few surviving copies (www.roseankhpublishing.com) as well as an online historical archive dedicated to the Alexandrian witchcraft tradition (www. alexandrianwitchcraft.org).

Also by Rose Ankh Publishing

Magic: A Life in More Worlds than One by David Conway

Born to be King: A Glimpse Into the Apprenticeship of the Witch and Magician by Alex Sanders

Forthcoming – a selection:

The Cryptographic Code of
Ancient Sacred Literature or
Truth Lost and Found
by Lt. Colonel George Close L. H.

Magic: A Life in More Worlds
than One
by David Conway – Deluxe,
Limited Edition

Magic: A Return to More Worlds
than One (working title)
by David Conway

Secret Wisdom
by David Conway,
Revised Edition

The Ecstatic Mother Portrait
of Maxine Sanders - Witch Queen
by Richard Deutch,
with commentary by Maxine Sanders

King of the Witches: The World of
Alex Sanders by June Johns,
with commentary by Maxine Sanders

Flame Beneath the Cauldron
(working title)
by Len Roberts

*Born to be King: A Glimpse Into
the Apprenticeship of the Witch and
Magician Alex Sanders* – Deluxe,
Limited Edition

The Alex Sanders Lectures
by Alex Sanders and others,
with commentary by Maxine Sanders